I0503846

Fatty Liver Diet

Treat, Reverse, and Cure Fatty Liver Disease One Bite at a Time

By

Dr. Junaid Tariq

Fatty Liver Diet

Copyright © 2019

All rights reserved. This book or any portion thereof may not be reproduced or used in any manner whatsoever without the express written permission of the publisher except for the use of brief quotations in a book review.

ISBN: 9781698218946

Warning and Disclaimer

Every effort has been made to make this book as accurate as possible. However, no warranty or fitness is implied. The information provided is on an "as-is" basis. The author and the publisher shall have no liability or responsibility to any person or entity with respect to any loss or damages that arise from the information in this book.

MEDICAL DISCLAIMER: The information available in this book is from my own personal research and it has not been endorsed by the medical field.

Publisher contact

Skinny Bottle Publishing

books@skinnybottle.com

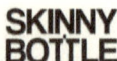

About the Author ix

Dr. Junaid Tariq ix

Chapter One... 11

Introduction 11

Now you'll be wondering what's all this fuss about?. 12

Chapter Two... 15

Anecdote.. 15

Chapter Three.. 18

Why is the Liver Important? 18

Chapter Four 21

Fatty Liver.. 21

Chapter Five 24

Causes Fatty liver and How to Diagnose it? 24

Lifestyle 24

Genetics 26

Gut Health Issues.. 28

Miscellaneous Causes... 29

Detection of Fatty Liver.. 30

Chapter Six.. 32

Can Diet Reverse Fatty Liver? 32

The Role of Triglycerides.. 33

The Role of Vegetable Oils..................................... 33

The Role of Choline 33

The Role of Saturated Fats................................34

Health Benefits of Various Foods.......................34

Cruciferous Vegetables.......................................34

Leafy Greens...35

Bitter Greens..35

Yogurt...35

Omega-3 Fatty Acid- Rich Foods.......................35

Foods with Vitamin C...36

Onions and Garlic...36

Hummus and Tahini...36

Olives..36

Eggs..36

Avocados...37

Chapter Seven..40

Ketogenic Diet Plan- The Basics........................40

"We're born in a state of ketosis".....................41

Why High Fat and Moderate Protein?...............43

Chapter Eight...44

Beginning a Ketogenic Diet Plan.......................44

Steps to Begin..44

Foods to Consume..45

Salads...46

Fibrous Vegetables...47

Fats to Use in Cooking.. 48

Fats for Cold Dressings... 48

Foods to Use in Limited.. 48

Beverages to Choose.. 49

Quick Snacks 49

Additional Tips.. 51

Chapter Nine 56

The Mediterranean Diet... 56

Constituents of the Mediterranean Diet................. 57

Fish... 57

Olive Oil.. 58

Legumes 58

Garlic 59

Capers 59

Chapter Ten.. 60

Following a Mediterranean Diet 60

Average Daily Intake... 60

Average Weekly Intake.. 61

Weekly Meal Plan 61

Quick Snacks 63

Chapter Eleven... 65

Liver Detox 65

Chapter Twelve... 68

Beginning a Fatty Liver Detox..68

  Breakfast..68

  Lunch and Dinner 70

  Lunch Ideas 70

  Chapter Thirteen..75

Salads to Detox Fatty Liver..75

  Spinach Salad..75

  Beet Salad..76

  Mushroom and Avocado Salad...............................77

  Marinated Vegetarian Asian-style Salad................78

  Salad Dressings..79

  Hummus..80

  Chapter Fourteen..82

Detox Soups for Fatty Liver..82

  Liver Cleansing Soup 82

  Lentil Soup..83

  Tomato Soup...85

  Traditional Chicken Soup 85

  Chapter Fifteen...88

Other Foods for Fatty Liver Detox 88

  Quick Snacks 88

  Low-Carbohydrate Ice-cream................................89

  Raw Juices...90

Liver Cleansing Juice..90

Liver Tonic Juice...91

Fatty Liver Juice...91

Tips to Dine Out...92

Thai, Chinese, and Vietnamese Cuisine 92

Italian Cuisine..92

French Cuisine..93

Japanese Cuisine...93

Middle-Eastern Cuisine 93

Indian Cuisine..93

Café Cuisines 94

Detox Super Foods..94

Chapter Sixteen...96

Simplifying your Fatty Liver Diet...96

Prohibited Foods...96

Shopping Tips...97

Vital Principles you Should Never Forget.....................98

Chapter Seventeen 113

Conclusion 113

About the Author

Dr. Junaid Tariq

Backed by 10-years of academic learning and 4 years of research career in medical sciences, I now work as a medical, health and nutrition writer and scientific consultant. My writing is always based on current evidence informed by peer-reviewed journal articles, government and peak health body guidelines, and medical experts, irrespective of the target audience.

My professional focus is on all-natural nutrition and attainable, healthy physiques. I believe that in the modern world when scientists have discovered cures for almost all ailments, there is still no substitute for nature.

Malikjunaidtariq@gmail.com

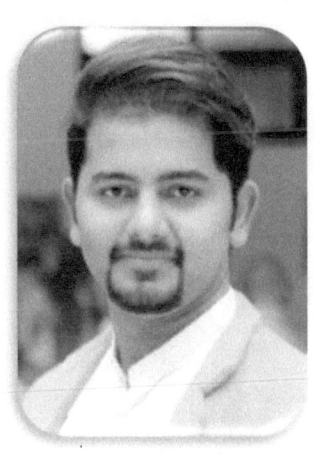

JUNAID TARIQ

Chapter One

Introduction

A sedentary lifestyle has become a common way of living. If you follow the lifestyle of a typical American then most probably you've seen your fair share of formidable plates. Your breakfast would start with a bowl full of sugary cereal or stacked up pancakes drenched in maple-flavored syrup. As soon as you finish breakfast, you've already set your habits for high obesity states.

Now that you're started gaining weight, you'd be wondering where the fat would hit you first. Is it going to be your Heart? Vessels? Kidneys? Pancreases? Or maybe it's going to be fat thighs- your worst nightmare? WRONG!

The liver- one of the most underrated organs of the human body- is a nutrient processing factory. It is possibly the largest internal organ of our body, nearly the size of a football, and located in the upper right area of the abdomen, just beneath the diaphragm. In a healthy adult, the liver weighs about 3 pounds.

Receiving almost 30% of the total blood circulating in the circulatory system every second, the liver performs over 500 different functions. It generates a total of 13,000 different chemical agents and maintains approximately 2000 internal systems of enzymes. Additionally, the liver also supports the functionality of almost every other organ in some facet.

We all know that carbohydrates are important sources of energy, but it is our liver that actually manages to release the energy trapped inside these carbohydrates. It works as a fat processing factory by breaking down 80% of the total cholesterol and phospholipid content to store them as a backup energy source. Blood proteins and clotting proteins are also the products generated by a healthy liver. Our liver filters blood normalizes blood sugar makes bile, detoxifies the body, and regulates hormones.

Now you'll be wondering what's all this fuss about?

Did you ever wonder what would happen if we ever lose this handy organ? Losing a liver can cause death within 24 hours as some of the most crucial life processes are entirely dependent on the liver!

While we acknowledge its effect on the heart and the circulatory system, we often tend to forget how it can deteriorate the liver. The excess calorie intake and a lack of exercise contribute to the buildup of fat in the liver, hindering its functionality. The damage does not remain limited to the liver itself but starts disturbing other organs of the body as well.

Before moving ahead, ask yourself these questions.

• Do you often feel tired or fatigued?

• Do you feel discomfort or pain in your back, abdomen or lower torso?

• Do you often feel nauseous?

• Have you completely lost your appetite?

• Do your skin and eyes look pale and yellow?

• Are you a binge drinker? Do you consume alcohol on a regular basis?

• Are you obese or fighting to shed extra pounds?

• Have you noticed any patches of discoloration around your neck or underarms?

• Do you often struggle with skin problems and do not know the reason?

• Do you feel cramping in the abdominal area?

• Do you suffer from confusion or headaches? Does concentrating and making judgments difficult for you lately?

• Are you always hungry? Do you constantly rely on starchy or sugary food as snacks?

If you have answered yes to most of the questions above then, boy, I've some bad news for you. These symptoms depict that you have got more than just fat thighs to work on.

Despite being a significant health concern, no medication has proven to be effective in treating fatty liver disease. Because the fatty liver is mostly secondary to other diseases, the treatment revolves around addressing the primary issues. Obesity is the biggest factor of fatty liver and the primary basis of its treatment.

Fighting obesity and reducing weight can be hard, but with the selection of the right food and nutrition, fatty liver can be cured easily. The focus of the book will be on the importance of diet and nutrition for curing fatty liver. Being the only treatment option for fatty liver, the right kind of diet can completely reverse the liver damage and restore the normal functionality of the liver.

Chapter Two

Anecdote

"You can't control everything in life, but you can control what you put in your body"

Miracles happen. That's how Samuel, one of my patients, survived a progressive case of fatty liver. When 46-year-old Samuel started experiencing bouts of stomach pain right before Christmas, he brushed it off as a cause of too much indulgence in the pre-holiday celebrations. Things got a lot worse when he suddenly started vomiting blood.

Because Samuel was a food lover and loved eating, his first guess was stomach ulcers. Samuel was probably eating spicier and unhealthy food, which also explains his obesity. However, many scans, tests, and biopsies later, he was shocked to learn the source of his pain: fatty liver. His liver had accumulated so much fat in its cells that it was actually failing. His liver enzymes were constantly elevated and failed to normalize even after proper medical treatment.

The condition of his liver was so bad that most of my colleagues predicted how a liver transplant would be crucial to keep Samuel alive, but for me, this wasn't the end. "Looking at a life with a failed liver, it just isn't a possibility," was the first thing he expressed. That's when I realized, "something extraordinary had to be done". Something that no medicine can accomplish and no procedure can fix.

Clearly, obesity was the biggest factor jeopardizing his liver health. For a long time, Samuel had wondered why the 'switch' in his mind wasn't turned on to healthy eating and natural management of his obesity. He had read a lot of books, listened to podcasts and tried to develop an understanding why he made poor choices about what to eat while he was fully aware of the consequences. Samuel expressed how he was not able to exercise on a regular basis because of his tight job schedule.

I decided to seal the fate of his fatty liver disease with the help of diet and nutrition.

Each week, Samuel attended a three-hour-long session where he learned about a number of topics- how to read food labels, organic versus non-organic food, food sensitivities, anti-inflammatory diets, blood sugar, the significance of dietary fiber, keto diet, environmental influences on food, and a lot more.

I made sure that Samuel controlled his dietary habits and chose the most suitable diet plans throughout his journey towards recovery. The right kinds of foods and diet schedules started doing the magic, shortly after which I began noticing a significant level of changes in Samuel. He lost weight, overcame most of the symptoms of fatty liver, and improved the overall quality of life.

"I think my success can be credited to sticking to the right kind of nutrition and diet chart. Everything feels completely different this time – I'm motivated to achieve overall good health, and overcoming fatty liver is just an aspect of that", says Samuel who has lost a significant amount of weight and has successfully beaten fatty liver by just modifying his everyday eating habits.

In my opinion, our health care system has failed when a doctor fails to treat an illness that is treatable. Fatty Liver has no medical cure, but If Samuel can do it, so can you.

"All it takes to cure a fatty liver is motivation and the right kind of diet."

Chapter Three

Why is the Liver Important?

You often hop around the gym to get rid of the excess belly fat; you frequently visit the dentist just to gloss up the teeth and go to all the healthcare facilities to treat different organs of your body. During all this hassle, you tend to forget the most important organ of the body- the liver.

"Your liver is different from other organs as it cannot be compensated by other systems or machines."

Physically positioned in the upper right quadrant of the abdomen, it serves as a site for the most vital processes of the human body. The liver cells, also known as hepatocytes, play an important role in the maintenance of normal hepatic functions such as metabolic regulation. All the complex chemical processes taking place in your body are collectively termed as metabolism. This includes the hematological metabolism and the metabolism of everything you consume including fats, carbohydrates, and proteins.

As you consume carbohydrates, the liver processes them to derive most of the glucose content from them. This glucose content is stored in the liver cells in the form of glycogen. The liver can release this stored glycogen whenever the body demands it, for example when the body is constantly fasting. Additionally, when the body is starving, the liver activates a series of processes that convert the protein content of your body into glucose to fulfill the needs. This sufficiently explains the role of the liver in maintaining the levels of blood glucose.

In a similar mechanism, the liver also serves a primary role in fat metabolism. It produces lipoprotein lipase which is essential to transport fats, triglycerides, and cholesterol from one part of the body to another. The liver provides a site for protein metabolism to take place. It allows the joining of different amino acids to form proteins necessary for survival. Some of these proteins include clotting factors and albumin. Not only does the liver regulates the proteins, fats, and carbohydrates in your body, it also aids in hematological regulation which is a process through which the liver controls the composition of blood. It regulates the concentration of chemicals in blood and breaks down its nutrient content to allow ease of usage.

One of the most important and well-known functions of the liver is perhaps, the production of bile. Bile is a yellowish fluid with alkaline pH produced by healthy hepatocytes. It consists of 85% of water and 10% of bile salts. Bile salts are fat emulsifiers and are required for the normal absorption and digestion of the fats. Bile also takes part in the detoxification process in which the toxic substances such as drugs, circulating in the body as a byproduct of metabolic products, are removed via feces. The hepatocytes produce bile and secrete them into tiny tubes that join together to develop into bile ductules and eventually open in the gallbladder. Within the gallbladder, the bile remains stored until it is required in the small intestine for the absorption of fat.

The liver is also a storehouse of vitamins and nutrients including vitamin-B12, Vitamin D, Vitamin A, copper, and iron. It also takes part in the secretion of angiotensinogen, an agent that acts on the kidneys to regulate blood pressure. It also transfers over 75% of the total blood around the body.

Chapter Four

Fatty Liver

"You cannot replicate liver functions by dialysis and certainly cannot insert a pacemaker to increase its efficiency."

Fatty liver is a chronic disease that has been plaguing society for the past decades. This disease has spread internationally affecting individuals belonging to different areas of the world. It is, thankfully, a reversible condition in which fats in the form of triglycerides within the liver cells. The disease can have multiple causes but on the basis of its two major risk factors, it is classified into two subtypes.

Non-alcohol fatty liver disease (NAFLD) is a form of fatty liver disorder that is not associated with heavy use of alcohol. This is a chronic problem that is usually associated with obesity. Due to a rise in obesity among the

21

youth today, NAFLD has become a silent killer. The disease is simply characterized by fat in the liver with little or no presence of damage or inflammation.

On the other hand, the alcoholic fatty liver disease has strong ties to alcohol consumption. The liver is responsible for breaking down the majority of alcohol that you consume in order to remove it. However, this process can also cause the generation of several harmful substances. These substances damage the liver cells, induce inflammation, and interfere with the body's natural defense system. The alcoholic fatty liver disease is one of the earliest forms of alcohol-related liver diseases, the next ones being alcoholic hepatitis and liver cirrhosis.

"The rule of this disease is simple; the more alcohol you consume, the more you harm your liver."

The accumulation of fat in both types of fatty liver is sometimes accompanied by a progressive inflammatory condition of the liver, known as Steatohepatitis. Depending upon the type of underlying fatty liver disease, this may be termed as alcoholic steatohepatitis or non-alcoholic steatohepatitis. This condition can inflame the liver cells, initiate fibrosis, and may even lead to permanent scarring of the liver.

Sometimes, fatty liver can also be associated with other diseases that control fat metabolism. When the fat metabolism is interrupted, fats start to accumulate in the liver, precipitating the disease. Generally, it is very difficult to distinguish alcoholic fatty liver disease from NAFLD as both include micro-vascular and macro-vascular fatty abnormalities at various stages.

Steatosis is a relatively common disorder, affecting about 25 to 35% of the general population in the United States. Steatohepatitis may or may not be related to alcohol and the consequent damage. About 15.3 million people in the United States abuse alcohol or are completely dependent on it. Fatty liver is high expected to occur in 90 to 100% of these alcoholic abusers. Non-alcoholic steatohepatitis is detected in 1.2 to 9 percent of the patients that undergo routine liver biopsy.

NAFLD, on the other hand, is detectable in more than 80% of obese individuals. More than half of the patient's schedules for bariatric surgery also have non-alcoholic steatohepatitis. On an international scale, 46.5% of alcoholics consuming more than 60 g of alcohol per day have this disease in comparison with 94% of the alcoholics with underlying obesity.

Fatty liver can occur in all age groups. In the case of alcoholic steatosis, the condition may worsen with age. This is because of the increased organ susceptibility and the fact that the liver starts handling alcohol differently as a person ages.

"In adolescents of the United States, NAFLD is considered to be the most common liver disease."

Non-alcoholic steatohepatitis is the third most common cause of liver diseases in adults of the U.S. It is also a primary reason for elevated transaminases levels and is found to recur within 6 months of having a liver transplant.

I bet the statistics have already got you worried!

Chapter Five

Causes Fatty liver and How to Diagnose it?

For the detection of fatty liver, it is important to identify the risk factors that may trigger the onset of this disease. Alcoholism is a basic risk factor for alcoholic fatty liver disease. Men who consume more than four pints or eight units of alcohol and women who drink five units of it on a daily basis are more likely to develop this disorder.

In addition to alcohol consumption, several other important factors can also lead to the development of fatty liver.

Lifestyle

"Studies have proven that sitting for only 2 hours right after having a meal can reduce insulin sensitivity and

can increase the levels of blood sugar, predisposing to fatty liver."

Lifestyle is said to greatly accelerate the development of fatty liver. Overeating, paired with a sedentary life, primarily contributes to the progression of this disease.

Insulin resistance is commonly observed as a side effect of eating too much and not exercising at all. It is also one of the main reasons why fats begin to accumulate in the liver. Within the body, insulin resistance initiates the release of fatty acids from the fat cells, and sugar begins to develop in the blood. The excessive amount of sugar and fatty acids; both from the diet and blood, make their way to the liver and are converted to fat and then stored in the hepatocytes.

As long as the muscles, liver, and adipose cells remain resistant to insulin, the loading of sugar in the blood and the accumulation of fat in the liver will continue to occur. This turns into a vicious cycle that keeps repeating itself to exacerbate the state of the fatty liver.

Eating a lot of sugar and fat allows the cell to fill up with energy. At some point, the level of energy becomes so high that the cells fail to respond to insulin. Under such circumstances, the liver has to receive all excessive sugars and fats and to store it in its cells in order to save the body from the destructive impacts of high levels of sugar and fat in the blood.

The fastest way in which you can increase the fat build-up is by eating too many carbohydrates. Fructose, in particular, causes fat accumulation in the liver. This is an important aspect since the control of fatty liver through diet rests around this concept.

Observing a sedentary lifestyle can also make your body cells respond less to insulin. Imagine what will happen to your body if you keep sitting most of the time sitting while most of the meals you are consuming are overloaded with fats and carbohydrates.

This is the reason why the majority of the researchers agree upon the fact that improvement of insulin sensitivity can essentially treat fatty liver disease.

Genetics

Like a lot of other diseases, fatty liver disease is polygenic in nature. This means that specific genes and the interactions occurring between them can increase or decrease the susceptibility of a person towards the development of fatty liver.

One of the genetic variants is of particular importance in this regard. The variant is known as PNPLA3 I148M and is highly associated with the development of fatty liver. This does not even require the presence of other problems such as insulin resistance, dyslipidemia, diabetes, or even obesity.

However, this does not mean that the presence of genes means you are definitely going to suffer from this disease. For instance, the PNPLA3 I148M gene variant can cause the progression of the disease only in the combination of other factors such as unhealthy dietary patterns, alcohol abuse, inactivity, viral infection, and a high amount of fructose.

The fact that fatty liver disease is polygenic in nature provides a justification for why fatty liver disease tends to exist in clusters within different families. This is the reason why it is extremely important to adopt an extremely healthy lifestyle if your ancestors have been struggling with this particular disease.

Other genetic factors may also impact your likelihood of developing this disease. These factors may include ethnicity and gender and this can affect the likelihood of developing fatty liver disease. Some older studies have also found that women are naturally more susceptible to developing this disease but now it is being said that it is more commonly seen in men.

Scientists have also postulated that the gender difference, in terms of fatty liver, is possibly due to the difference in fat distribution and the concentration of hormones. Men have more fat stored close to their organs which is the type of fat that is inflammatory. This pattern of fat deposition increases the risk of fatty liver and many other diseases in males. On the other hand, women are more likely to accumulate fat in thighs and hips which is less inflammatory as compared to males.

As far as ethnicity is concerned, studies have established that African Americans are exposed to the lowest risk of developing fatty liver in spite of the fact that they are highly exposed to the risk of developing type 2 diabetes. This difference is justified because of the different patterns of fat deposition too. In contrast to this, Hispanics and Asians seem to have the greatest risk of fatty liver disease. Scientists are of the belief that this is because these two ethnicities are more likely to store their fat in close proximity to organs.

It is important to mention here that other genes might also have certain effects on the development of fatty liver. These might not be your genes but the genes present in your microbiome.

Gut Health Issues

Your microbiome consists of over 100 trillion bacteria normally lining your gut. These different types of bacteria that keep flourishing and perishing from time to time have an important effect on your health, especially on the health of the liver.

Scientific studies focusing on the microbiome of different obese patients have established that such patients have a reduced amount of a particular type of bacteria. This particular bacterium is known as Bacteroidetes. At the same time, the levels of another bacteria known as Firmicutes are found to be increased. This disturbance in the ratio of these two species of bacteria causes an increase in the absorption of lipopolysaccharides.

What are these lipopolysaccharides? These are components that are found in the cell membranes of most gram-negative bacterial species such as Bacteroidetes. However, these components are not harmful. Lipopolysaccharides are, in fact, endotoxins that stimulate a strong inflammatory response within the body. This helps to contribute to the development of insulin resistance in the liver and leads to obesity.

The microbiome of every person is unique. However, it has become quite clear about the source which generates this obesity-inducing microbiome. The source is a diet that causes the development of obesity, more specifically, a diet rich in sugar and fat Consuming a diet high in fat and sugar causes a reduction in the microbiome diversity and disturbs Firmicutes-to-Bacteroidetes ratio. This will result in the development of obesity-causing microbiome profiles that favors the progression of fatty liver disease.

Moreover, the increase in the absorption of lipopolysaccharide due to the consumption of poor diet and an obesity-causing microbiota can disturb the liver functions so much that fatty acid may even progress to steatohepatitis.

Miscellaneous Causes

Various hereditary problems like hemochromatosis, Wilson's disease, Alagille syndrome, galactosemia, type 1 storage disease, and alpha-1 antitrypsin deficiency can naturally predispose a person to a higher risk of developing fatty liver.

People who are already suffering from some kind of autoimmune disorder are also susceptible to developing fatty liver disease. In such cases, the liver is already targeted for damage by the immune system and the development of fatty liver only makes things worse. In addition to this, disorders of the bile duct including primary sclerosing cholangitis, and primary biliary cirrhosis may also contribute to fatty liver.

In some cases, inhalation or ingestion of toxins can also precipitate fatty liver. The significance of toxic hepatitis is worth mentioning in this regard. Consuming certain drugs, including both prescription and over-the-counter medications, can sometimes lead to severe reactions, consequently developing fatty liver. People who are already infected with viruses, such as hepatitis A, B or C virus are more likely to develop fatty liver.

Detection of Fatty Liver

Detection of fatty liver disease requires a thorough history, especially in reference to alcohol consumption. It is particularly important for determining the role of alcohol in the etiology of any abnormalities in the liver tests. History taking may also involve the family members who may reveal the past-alcoholic problems associated with the patients. There is no specific method or test for ruling out the possibility of drug-related toxicity. However, enough information can be obtained by reviewing all the recent and old medications including the alternative treatments and over-the-counter drugs for evaluating the possible causes. Severe forms of the disease may manifest in the form of weakness, abdominal discomfort, nausea, and anorexia. Jaundice or yellowing of the skin is also visible in almost 15% of the individuals who are admitted to the hospital.

"NAFLD is asymptomatic most of the time."

However, upon questioning, most of the people suffering from the disease report malaise, persistent fatigue, and upper abdominal discomfort. In people having progressive forms of non-alcoholic steatohepatitis, other symptoms can also be present such as edema, ascites, and jaundice. Laboratory findings indicate an elevation in the serum alanine aminotransferases levels which ultimately leads to the successful detection of fatty liver disease. In NAFLD, hepatomegaly is a common sign. These patients are often tested positive for other conditions such as splenomegaly, angiomas, edema, ascites, varices, menstrual disorders, and gynecomastia if the disease has caused liver cirrhosis. The disease may also present itself in the form of dark skin discoloration. Patches of this discoloration are often present below the arms or on the neck.

Upon suspecting an incidence of fatty liver disease, several tests may also be performed including a blood test to confirm the liver profiles. CT scan or an MRI can also be used for imaging purposes. Lastly, a liver biopsy is often recommended in which a tissue sample is taken by inserting a long needle in the liver and taking out a bit of the organ for laboratory examinations.

Chapter Six

Can Diet Reverse Fatty Liver?

So, now you'll be asking, "What can I do to protect and heal 'my precious' liver?"

Welcome to a new world of answers!

There are a lot of speculations about the role of diet and nutrition in the progression of fatty liver disease. One of the common questions which might be asked by the patients is that can diet treat fatty liver?

The answer to this question is yes, and the reason is quite simple. Both types of fatty liver diseases occur due to alteration in fat metabolism and this is something we can control through diet.

To understand this better, it is important to analyze how imbalanced nutrition can lead to the development of fatty liver.

The Role of Triglycerides

Most of the time, a high triglyceride level in the blood is due to high carbohydrate consumption, particularly the consumption of fructose. The elevated triglyceride levels are a consequence of consuming a diet rich in carbohydrates. It has also been proven that the consumption of fructose in high amounts increases the blood pressure, elevates the triglyceride levels and causes inflammation and insulin resistance within the liver.

The Role of Vegetable Oils

Consuming high levels of vegetable oil is also associated with the development of fatty liver. This is because vegetable oils naturally contain higher levels of omega-6 polyunsaturated fats having pro-inflammatory effects. Sometimes, these oils are hydrogenated, causing the development of trans-fat in them which are particularly dangerous for the liver. Some of these oils include corn oil, soya bean oil, and canola oils.

The Role of Choline

Choline is an essential nutrient required for normal transportation of fats out of the liver. The lack of choline has been found to result in liver damage. Fatty liver, particularly, NAFLD, can be cured by the simple addition of this dietary nutrient. This factor seems to be dominant over the other dietary factors including sugar, fat, and even alcohol. The high significance of choline in treating fatty liver is backed up by science but has not been able to enter into the mainstream consciousness.

The Role of Saturated Fats

It is important to clarify here that not all fats are your enemy. Saturated fats, in fact, helps the liver to shed excess fat in as little as three days, according to science. Saturated fat has also been found to reverse alcohol-related injury in the liver. So, instead of focusing on a carbohydrate-rich diet, a simple alteration to consuming saturated fats can make a lot of difference.

Diet is indeed important for controlling and reversing fatty liver irrespective of its cause. Following an accurate diet plan will not only improve the health of your liver but will also enhance the quality of life.

Health Benefits of Various Foods

It is important for you to know about the benefits of certain foods so that you might be able to incorporate them into your daily diet.

Cruciferous Vegetables

These vegetables have a high level of mineral sulfur which enhances the process of liver detoxification. Cruciferous vegetables include Brussels sprouts, broccoli, cabbage, broccolini, and cauliflower.

Leafy Greens

Dark, leafy green vegetables have high levels of chlorophyll and vitamin K, both extremely important for general health. Leafy green vegetables include bok choy, boakk choy, mustard greens, spinach, watercress, silverbeet, choy sum, and other Asian greens.

Bitter Greens

Bitter greens such as endive, radicchio, rocket, and chicory enhance the flow of bile.

Yogurt

Yogurt consists of certain friendly bacteria. Be sure to use plain, full-fat yogurt with no sweetener or try Greek-style yogurt.

Omega-3 Fatty Acid- Rich Foods

Omega-3 fatty acids are required for the maintenance of healthy cell membranes. They can also be used to decrease the inflammation of the liver cells often seen in the fatty liver. Omega-3 fatty acids can be found in sardines, salmon, tuna, mackerel, trout, hemp, flaxseeds, chia seeds, walnuts, and grass-fed lambs.

Foods with Vitamin C

Vitamin C particularly improves the function of the liver. The best sources for getting this vitamin are limes, lemons, oranges, grapefruits, kiwi fruit, mandarins, berries, tomatoes, and capsicums.

Onions and Garlic

Both onion and garlic consist of certain cleansing products that purify the liver and blood. It should ideally be eaten on a regular basis. The raw form is preferable but can be used in the cooked form.

Hummus and Tahini

Tahini and hummus both are rich sources of minerals, calcium in particular. They also have high amounts of healthy fats.

Olives

Both forms of olives i.e. green and black consist of antioxidants and healthy fats.

Eggs

Eggs have a good amount of sulfur and protein. They are healthy for the liver and will not affect the cholesterol levels. Eggs are particularly useful if you are trying to lose weight and reverse fatty liver.

Avocados

Avocados have high levels of vitamin E as compared to other food items. They are extremely healthy for liver health.

Now, before heading towards different ways, let's take a look at how an appropriate diet can bear fruit for you:

• Your liver will naturally dissolve all the fat which will be safely flushed out of the body. This will automatically lower the risk of severe complications such as liver cirrhosis and liver cancer.

• Your belly fat will reduce and thighs will shrink as the liver restores its function and the body normalizes its hormone levels

• You will feel that your skin is getting softer and blemishes are clearing up. The skin will begin to look a lot younger since all the poisons irritating it will be flushed out. Other skin diseases such as dermatitis, psoriasis, and eczema will start to heal and even dissipate on their own as the liver gets healthy again.

• You will feel sharpness in your concentration and focus because your brain will no longer be filled with acidic blood having toxic effects. The level of alertness will increase and you will be able to think more clearly.

• You will feel a noticeable difference in the vision, especially in low light. This will make it easier for you to perform certain tasks such as driving at night. Colors will seem more vibrant. If you have weak eyesight, you may not even need as strong a prescription.

• You will begin to sleep better without the help of drugs. You will be well-rested and ready to make every single day count.

• You will notice a reduction in bowel and stomach problems because of liver aids in digestion. Fats, toxins, and sugars will start eliminating through your perfectly healthy digestive system at a faster pace. At the same time, important minerals and nutrients will be maximally absorbed to help you thrive.

• You will notice yourself getting out of the depression and anger that have become a permanent part of your life due to constant liver illness. There will be a significant reduction in stress and mood swings as well.

And of course, there will be many improvements that you can't visualize but can certainly feel are happening nevertheless:

• You will extend your life for many years, perhaps even decades.

• You will be reducing your chance of getting serious diseases such as cirrhosis, heart attacks, and even cancer.

• You will decrease the possibility of other diseases like arthritis, diabetes, and digestive problems.

Now that you know that nutrition can control fatty liver, it's time to know about the right kind of diet plans to move ahead and combat the disease.

Chapter Seven

Ketogenic Diet Plan- The Basics

The benefits of a ketogenic diet are far-stretching. A ketogenic diet tends to improve your overall health with the help of a metabolic switch present in the primary cellular fuel source. Your body, as well as your brain, are adapted to this cellular fuel source which is normally considered to have carbohydrate-based fuels. Glucose is considered as the energy currency in your body which is normally derived from starch and other sugars. In a ketogenic diet, this fuel source is switched from the carbohydrate-derived glucose to fat-derived ketones.

To understand how the ketogenic diet works against fatty liver, it is important to know what ketogenesis and ketosis are. Ketogenesis is a metabolic process whereas ketosis is a body state, both of which form the basis of the ketogenic diet. Ketosis is a metabolic pathway in which your body starts utilizing ketones instead of glucose to form energy.

This means that it does not need to rely on carbohydrates and sugar anymore. Humans developed an ability to burn ketones during times when food was unavailable to them, thereby; adopting a natural tendency for ketosis. This principle can be used in patients with fatty liver to help them get rid of excess fat and repair the damaged organ side by side. As it is said,

"We're born in a state of ketosis"

Various studies have been performed on the effect of ketosis in relation to diseases. Ketone bodies have been found to exert some extremely beneficial impacts on the human body and the elevation in the levels of these ketone bodies has been favored as a treatment regimen for a number of diseases. The main reason for this is because ketones can significantly improve the functionality of the cellular energy pathways. Moreover, they can also improve the mitochondrial health of hepatic cells. The ketogenic diet is, therefore, being used to improve the states of epilepsy, diabetes, cancer, Alzheimer's disease, and even autism.

There are different ways of implementing a ketogenic diet plan with low carbohydrate content. However, a diet containing a higher amount of fat, moderate levels of protein and low carbohydrates is the preferable one.

There are many ways of implementing a low carbohydrate, ketogenic diet plans but most involve following a higher fat, moderate protein, low carb food plan. Most people have misconceptions that a ketogenic diet involves a high amount of protein intake but this is not true. There are differences between a ketogenic diet and a general low-carb diet, with the main differences lying in the amounts of proteins and carbohydrates taken on a daily basis.

• A ketogenic diet involves keeping a track of carbohydrate levels in all the foods being eaten. It requires you to bring down your daily carbohydrate intake to as low as 20 to 60 grams per day. For some people, keeping the daily carbohydrate intake below 100 grams may also work, but for the majority, this level is not sufficient to initiate ketosis. In addition to this, the daily protein requirement must be dependent on the lean body mass or the ideal body weight. Protein take also vary according to the gender, height, and amount of physical activity of each person. Eating a high level of protein can disturb the process of ketosis, so it is important to keep a check on the daily protein intake as well.

• The nutrient intake during a ketogenic diet can be distributed into three separate means i.e. calories taken from fat, protein, and carbohydrates. When calories are not restricted, a70 to 75% of them are derived from fat and 20 to 25% from protein. Carbohydrates only account for 5 to 10% of the total calorie intake on a daily basis. Although calorie counting is not required during a ketogenic diet, it is important to know how the percentages of macronutrients can be impacted by calorie intake. Extremely low or extremely high levels of calories can alter the percentages of macronutrients and it is important to keep this point in mind throughout the course of the ketogenic diet.

The key concept in the implementation of a ketogenic diet is to always keep in mind that your primary goal is to replace carbohydrate-containing food with fatty foods while maintaining a moderate protein consumption side by side.

Why High Fat and Moderate Protein?

One of the most frequently asked questions by the users is that why should you take a diet high in fat but moderate in terms of proteins? This is because fats have minimal or no effect on blood sugar levels and insulin concentration. Protein, on the other hand, can affect both of these factors to a great extent. If you consume high levels of proteins for your lean muscle mass (more than 1.5 grams per kg of lean body mass), it can trigger gluconeogenesis and elevate the blood sugar levels.

Consumption of proteins can also increase insulin levels in the blood on a temporary basis. The raised insulin levels can consequently interfere with the normal production of ketone bodies and disrupt the foundation of the ketogenic diet.

Chapter Eight

Beginning a Ketogenic Diet Plan

The ketogenic diet plan can vary from person to person depending upon a number of factors.

Steps to Begin

To prepare a custom ketogenic plan, follow these simple steps:

Calculate your ideal body weight. You can either use a calculator or mark the target on your own.

Mark your daily caloric intake. Keep in mind that this calorie requirement has to be according to your weight requirement. Try using a calorie calculator to find out the number of calories you require according to your BMI.

Evaluate the number of macronutrients. Figure out how much fat, carbohydrates, and proteins do you consume on a daily basis. You can then use software to keep a track of your numbers more efficiently.

A ketogenic diet requires you to consume proteins in an amount of 1 to 1.5 grams per kilogram of lean body mass.

In the case of carbohydrates, the aim is to stay below 60 grams each day, but this may vary. If you exercise on a daily basis and have a lot of muscle mass, you can eat more than that. In case you are diabetic or suffer from any other metabolic issues, the carbohydrate might require further reduction. If the weight loss is still not occurring, lower the carb intake even below 30 grams.

Calories coming from oils and fats are usually calculated after subtraction of the calories coming from carbohydrates and proteins.

Foods to Consume

It is always better to eat the foods recommended later in the diet plan. If you decide to eat other foods, do not forget to check their labels for total carbohydrate levels. Remember that the meat or dairy items must have less than 2 grams of carbohydrates and 5 grams in case of vegetables.

Select from the following foods to eat when you are hungry.

• Meat: lamb, goat, beef. Prefer grass-fed meat.

• Pork: pork loin, pork chops, Boston butt, ham, with no added sugars.

- Poultry: turkey, chicken, duck, pheasant, quail, goose.

- Wild-caught seafood: anchovies, cod, catfish, halibut, mahi-mahi, scrod, tuna, snapper, mackerel, flounder, and tuna. (Avoid fried or breaded seafood)

- Canned salmon and tuna can be consumed after checking for added sugars.

- Shellfish: lobster, clams, shrimps, oysters, squid, scallops, and mussels.

- Soy product including edamame, tofu, and tempeh after carefully checking the labels.

- Bacon and sausage with carbohydrate count less than 2g per serving.

- Avoid foods having whey protein.

- Whole eggs can be eaten in different forms such as deviled, hard-boiled, fried, poached, omelets, and scrambled.

Be sure not to use any breading, flour, or cornmeal.

One or two cups of salads and fibrous vegetables are inevitable on a daily basis.

One or two cups of salads and fibrous vegetables are inevitable on a daily basis.

Salads

Add the following vegetables to your salad greens:

- Cabbage

- Greens of all varieties
- Lettuce
- Parsley
- Chard
- Kale
- Spinach

Fibrous Vegetables

Mix and match from the following vegetables as per your liking,

- Bean sprouts and alfalfa
- Okra
- Rhubarb
- Broccoli
- Bell peppers
- Asparagus
- Bamboo shoots
- Radishes
- Mushrooms
- Cucumber
- Jicama
- Zucchini
- Water Chestnuts
- Sprouts

- Turnips

In the case of fats, minimizing vegetable oils and focusing on saturated animal fats are recommended

Fats to Use in Cooking

- Organic duck fat
- Organic olive oil
- Organic Lard
- Beef tallow
- Organic chicken fat
- Low-temperature frying in butter
- Organic coconut oil or cream concentrate
- Ghee

Fats for Cold Dressings

- Macadamia oil
- Avocado oil
- Seed and nut oil: sesame oil, almond oil, flaxseed oil, etc.
- Mayonnaise.

Foods to Use in Limited

The following foods have to be consumed in limited quantities on a daily basis:

- Dairy cream: up to 4 tablespoons
- Cheese: 4 ounces (avoid whipped, cream, and processed cheese)
- Olives: 7 a day
- Half an avocado
- Up to 4 tablespoons of mayonnaise
- Lime juice: 4 teaspoons
- Ketchup: 1 tablespoon of low sugar sauce only
- Soy sauce: 4 tablespoons
- 2 servings of sugar-free pickles

Beverages to Choose

- Decaf coffee
- Water
- Unsweetened almond milk (up to 2 cups a day)
- Flavored seltzer water
- Unsweetened herbal tea
- Clear Broth

Quick Snacks

- Hard-boiled eggs spread in mayonnaise or sour cream
- Make small pieces of cooked steak and add them to sour cream, cream cheese, or mayonnaise.

- Shrimp mixed with mayonnaise, minced onions and cucumber slices

- Beef jerky with no sugar

- Spread cheese and mayonnaise on a slice of turkey, ham, or salami and roll it up by itself

- Spread slices of smoked salmon with cream cheese and lemon juice

- Dip pork rinds into pesto sauce or ranch dressings

- Sugar-free pickles with cheddar cheese

- Stuff feta cheese in olives

- Roasted nuts

- Mix crab meat in lemon juice and cream cheese

- Stuff blue cheese mixture in celery

- Baked chicken wings with no breading

- Pork rinds with sour cream and low-carb salsa sauce

- Smoked salmon and scrambled eggs with cream cheese

- Cook bacon, mayonnaise, and tomato chunks in lettuce leaf

- Tuna in cream cheese and mayonnaise

- Fried Macadamia nuts in butter

- Slices of blue cheese with pecans

- Celery with a stuffing of almond butter

- Mix Greek yogurt with ginger, cardamom, sweetener, and cinnamon

- Take 2 ounces of heavy cream and cream cheese each and add sweetener

- Take one-fourth cup of almond butter and mix in heavy cream. Add a bit of sweetener

- Make antipasto using olives, peppers, salami, prosciutto, and cheese cubes

- Prepare crispy bacon and mix with sour cream and blue cheese. Add spice as per your requirement.

Additional Tips

You can follow the following tips to make the ketogenic diet more effective for your fatty liver disease.

1. Get a complete health checkup in addition to a blood panel test right before you are beginning to follow the diet plan. This will help you track the changes in your cholesterol, dietary habits, blood pressure, and other health parameters associated with fatty liver. Repeat these tests four to eight weeks later to check for any improvements.

2. Grab a carbohydrate counter guide as it will help you to learn and remember the carbohydrate count of different foods. Keeping a check on the carbohydrate count is a critical part of the ketogenic diet hence, it is important to develop an understanding of how to perform it accurately.

3. In order to stop unnecessary carbohydrate consumption, perform a carbohydrate sweep. This involves a thorough inspection of your kitchen cupboards and the fridge, removing everything containing high carb levels.

4. Once you have swiped your kitchen free, go shopping for new food. While you are on your trip, make sure to buy foods with extremely low carbohydrates.

5. Remember that the Ketogenic diet plan does not involve any special diet or food items. There is absolutely no need to buy any packaged food labeled as "low carbs". Ketogenic foods exist naturally and every whole food item which is closer to its natural state is essentially ketogenic. The only exception to this rule is the category consisting of artificial sweeteners. These sweeteners are highly processed but are necessary to include in the ketogenic diet program. This is because these artificial sweeteners tend to damage health lesser than the standard sugar found in sweetened food. Some people may prefer taking natural sugar alcohol sweeteners but these sweeteners are anti-ketogenic in nature can stop the process of ketosis in some individuals. So, it is better to test these sweeteners to check their effect on your overall health and weight.

6. Prepare yourself to spend more time in the kitchen. This is an important step to acknowledge as a ketogenic diet mostly involves self-cooking and eating what we call real foods. This would also be a great time to learn cooking if you are an amateur and you will gain experience about how to prepare low-carb food at home.

7.   Ponder over what meals you will cook and how would you like to do it. This step will help you to buy the right kind of food items and provide you with a framework to be followed when mealtime approaches. For example, if you are sure to pair some salmon with broccoli for dinner, it will help you to avoid choosing foods with high carbohydrates that you previously used to eat.

8.   An important tip for observing the ketogenic diet is to replace or modify your old habits. For example, if you went to a particular coffee place and had a bagel along with it, quit visiting the place. Start making coffee at home and cook some eggs as a snack.

9.   Maintain your hydration levels. As you lower your carbohydrate intake, the kidneys start excreting water. Much water is lost in this process and it may disturb the normal hydration of the body. So, make sure that you drink a sufficient level of water to replace what your kidneys are actively excreting. The rule of drinking 6 to 8 glasses of water can be applied here, however, I personally suggest drinking to the thirst. If you start suffering from muscle cramps and headaches, it is a sign that your body needs more water and salt.

10.   Avoid food that you know is loaded with carbohydrates. These are the foods that can drive your blood sugar and insulin levels. Cereal grains such as wheat are particularly toxic to people and have to be avoided strictly.

11.   Consider having natural supplements to fight certain issues that may appear in the ketogenic diet plan.

12.   You may need to buy ketosis test strips as these will help you to check and see if your body is favoring the process of ketosis. This is important to check during the first few weeks of starting a ketogenic diet. After 3 to 4 weeks, the body needs to become keto-adapted. Once the adaptation has occurred, the body starts burning ketones for getting energy. A blood ketone meter is also available in the market these days to keep a track of ketosis at home. This instrument is much more reliable and accurate.

13.   Devise a way to keep a track of your daily food intake and carbohydrate count. You can either make a spreadsheet, use any online food intake tracker, or simply make notes in your journal. Not only will this help you to keep on a line with respect to carbohydrates, but you will also have your own little book of personal experiences to look back to for guidance in case you go off-track.

14.   Do not forget to think about different social situations that you may have to encounter and think about how to handle them. These are the times when your temptations will be sky-touching and you can easily get blindsided by anyone. A casual hang out with friends can end up with nachos and fries. Remember to choose steak and salads instead.

15.   Do not focus on your weight fluctuations during the entire course of the ketogenic diet plan. Also, refrain from weighing yourself every day. Your weight can alter every day by 2 to 4 pounds, mostly because of the consumption and absorption of water. There is no way that you can keep a record of your daily fat loss in an accurate way, and

measuring weight, again and again, is just going to drive you crazy. Instead, focus on your long-term goal i.e. to get rid of fatty liver and all of its complications. Weigh yourself once every week or take body measurements if you are keen to track your progress. Better yet, just focus on the health benefits of this diet and the long-term changes in your health that this diet is going to bring. Knowing that your health is significantly improving is a strong reason to stick to the diet plan even if you do not notice any obvious change in your body or weight.

16.   Learn how to control your craving for sugar. You can try using different techniques and supplements that can aid you in overcoming the guilty thoughts of having a dessert or sipping on some soda. With the passage of time, you will realize that ketosis itself is a potent suppressor of appetite. This will make it easier for you to control your cravings later during your diet.

17.   Do not be scared of consuming high amounts of fat. There are different types of fats some of which are surprisingly helpful for your body. Take a closer look and observe the type of fats that you are consuming during a ketogenic diet plan. Choose natural and saturated fats such as olive oil and butter instead of seed-based vegetable oils.

Chapter Nine

The Mediterranean Diet

In an attempt to understand how the Mediterranean diet can help you with fatty liver, a simple rule is to be remembered i.e. "it is what the inside counts". The selection of herbs, beverages, and other food items included as a part of the Mediterranean diet are enriched with nutrients and phytonutrients that mainly cure your diseases and restore health. These nutrients bear benefits, ranging from antioxidant, anti-mutagenic, anti-inflammatory, antiviral, vasodilatory, and antithrombotic properties.

"Mediterranean diet consists of six important nutrients including carbohydrates, fat, protein, vitamins, water, and minerals."

By maintaining a balance between these essential nutrients, the Mediterranean diet will surely help you to lose fat and get rid of fatty liver along with all of its complications. In addition to these essential nutrients, the Mediterranean diet also promises to deliver phytonutrients, otherwise known as phytochemicals. These nutrients are not essential for the human body and if not taken, do not produce any deficiency. However, phytochemicals are extremely beneficial for health since their presence can improve the diet and help you fight diseases like fatty liver. Phytonutrients are typically found in plants and protect them from dangerous attacks of bugs, fungi, and other germs. More than 25,000 phytonutrients are currently found in the plants with a lot more on their way to discovery.

Constituents of the Mediterranean Diet

The question arises, what are the constituents of the Mediterranean diet that makes it different yet effective for treating fatty liver?

Fish

Fish is a source of two important fatty acids: omega-3, and omega-6 fatty acids. The ancient human diet used to contain both of these fatty acids in equal amounts. However, as time passed, the amount of omega-6 fatty acids increased to almost 20 times more than that of the omega-3 fatty acids. This is important to acknowledge because omega-3 fatty acids are of particular importance and their benefits cannot be replicated by any other type of fatty acids or supplements.

Extensive research has been performed on omega-3 fatty acids benefits. It has been proven to help protect the body from a number of cardiovascular complications, cancer, hypertension, arthritis, and depression. It also helps to relieve the signs of aging. Moreover, omega-3 fatty acids can also control obesity which is of particular importance in controlling fatty liver.

By choosing a Mediterranean diet, you are providing your body with high volumes of omega-3 fatty acids. Some sources of this particular fatty acids include bluefish, anchovy, herring, bluefish, sturgeon, mullet, and tuna, all of which are included in a Mediterranean diet plan.

Olive Oil

Olive oil is potentially rich in phytonutrients. These phytonutrients are known as phenolic antioxidants and are known to possess liver-protective functions. These can not only promote the general health of the liver but can also reverse any damage caused to it. Additionally, these phytonutrients also work as neuroprotective agents and help the body to fight against aging, Alzheimer's disease, spinal cord injury, Parkinsonism, and peripheral neuropathy.

Extra virgin olive oil and black olives are considered to have the highest amounts of phenolic antioxidants and can be used in moderation to control calories, reduce weight, and treat fatty liver all naturally.

Legumes

A variety of legumes including peas, green beans, soybeans, peanuts, chickpeas, alfalfa, lentils, dry beans, broad beans, and clover can be particularly useful in reversing fatty liver. All of them are included as a part of the Mediterranean diet. These legumes are also a rich source of phytonutrients that protect all the systems of the body from different diseases.

Garlic

Many people fail to realize the beneficial effects of garlic on general health. Like every other component of the Mediterranean diet, garlic also possesses high amounts of a phytonutrient named allicin. Allicin has antioxidant, antimicrobial and liver-protective properties and guarantees the complete restoration of health including reversal of fatty liver if used wisely.

Capers

The flower buds from this shrub are used in a lot of dishes including spaghetti puttanesca, chicken piccata, and eggplant caponata. However, very few people acknowledge the actual benefits of it. Research has proven that capers have anti-oxidative, antimicrobial, anti-inflammatory, anti-diabetic and immuno-modulatory properties that enhance the general health and make the body strong enough to fight diseases like fatty liver.

Chapter Ten

Following a Mediterranean Diet

The Mediterranean food pyramid serves as the best source for choosing what to eat and what to avoid. In simpler terms, food intake included in a Mediterranean diet can be divided into a daily and weekly schedule.

Average Daily Intake

- 2 to 3 servings of vegetables
- 4 to 6 servings of fruits
- Olive oil
- 1 to 2 glasses of wine
- Unrefined cereal and bread products
- 1 to 2 servings of low-fat dairy
- Frequent use of garlic, herbs, onions, and spices

Average Weekly Intake

- 4 to 5 servings of fish
- 4 to 5 servings of potato
- More than 4 servings of nuts, pulses, and olives
- 1 to 4 servings of eggs
- Moderate use of yogurt and cheese
- 1 to 3 servings of sweets (on a monthly basis)
- 4 to 5 servings of red meat and other meat products

If you are planning to try a Mediterranean diet, the following diet chart can be of considerable importance. Adjustments can be made regarding the food choices and the sizes of the portions.

Weekly Meal Plan

Monday

Breakfast: Consume Greek yogurt and add oats and strawberries.

Lunch: Prepare a whole grain sandwich using vegetables.

Dinner: Go for a tuna salad, using olive oil dressing. Consume a little piece of fruit as dessert.

Tuesday

Breakfast: Eat oatmeal with raisins.

Lunch: Consume the leftover tuna salad that you prepared last night

Dinner: Prepare a salad using olives, tomatoes, and feta cheese.

Wednesday

Breakfast: Cook omelet and add veggies such as tomatoes and onions. A piece of fruit can be eaten for a change of taste.

Lunch: Prepare a whole grain sandwich and add cheese and fresh vegetables.

Dinner: Go for Mediterranean lasagne.

Thursday

Breakfast: Consume yogurt with nuts. Add some sliced fruit.

Lunch: Eat the leftover lasagne from last night.

Dinner: Prepare broiled salmon and vegetables. Eat with brown rice

Friday

Breakfast: Throw in some eggs and vegetables and cook in olive oil

Lunch: Add strawberries, nuts, and oats in a Greek Yogurt.

Dinner: Cook grilled lamb and eat with baked potato and salad.

Saturday

Breakfast: Prepare oatmeal with raisins. Add some nuts and consume it with an apple.

Lunch: Eat a whole grain sandwich using vegetables.

Dinner: Bake a Mediterranean pizza using whole wheat. Use vegetables, cheese, and olives as toppings

Sunday

Breakfast: Omelet consisting of vegetables and olives.

Lunch: Eat the leftover pizza from the night before.

Dinner: Cook grilled chicken along with vegetables and potatoes. Consume fruit in place of dessert.

It is not necessary to keep a check on the calorie count. You also don't need to track the number of fats, proteins, and carbohydrates while following this diet plan.

Quick Snacks

A Mediterranean diet does not require you to eat more than three times a day. However, if you become hungry in between meal times, the following snacks can be tried:

- A few grapes or berries
- A small piece of fruit
- Baby carrots
- Greek yogurt
- Leftover food from the night before
- A few nuts
- Apple slices with almond butter

Chapter Eleven

Liver Detox

Liver detox is controversial as doctors generally say, "you can't detox your mighty liver as it already detoxifies itself".

This can be true, but taking into consideration the fact that fatty liver results in a toxin overload, the toxins which were actually meant to break down. But the deposited fats won't let the liver do its function. The health and well-being of every individual are dependent on the detoxification processes going on in their bodies. These processes are essential for the removal of harmful substances which can otherwise interfere with the normal functionality of different organ systems. Due to a high exposure rate to toxic care products, environmental pollution, and processed food, detox is required by most people.

Detoxification of the liver is also particularly helpful in the case of fatty liver. The liver, in this case, has lost its full capacity to work and requires a fresh start. Detoxification can successfully provide this fresh start to the liver. The process is similar to tuning up the car and cleaning out its spark plug that accelerates its performance and boosts the functions. In a similar way, by committing yourself to a healthy diet, you are actually supporting your body's detoxification systems and reducing their exposure to dangerous substances.

Detoxification of liver or liver cleanse is definitely not easy. You will often feel hungry and may suffer from weakness. However, it is not something that's impossible. There are a number of cleansing diets that can help with fatty liver but all of them seem to follow the same pattern. In a liver cleansing diet, you are required to give up all the unhealthy foods. It incorporates the use of juice or special tea for a given period of time, lasting 10 days to the maximum.

"The elimination of unhealthy foods and restriction of the daily food intake can help the liver purge itself and the body of all the toxic and harmful substances."

This can particularly be helpful in the case of fatty liver when abnormalities in liver functions have caused toxic agents to accumulate, further exacerbating the condition. Most of the people will discourage you from the side effects associated with liver cleansing diets. These side effects may include low blood sugar, low energy, fatigue, muscle aches, dizziness, and nausea. It is not wrong that following such a diet can lead to some alterations in your normal routine but the idea that a liver detox is harmful to your overall health is fundamentally wrong. This is because the diet can be altered and changed according to individual needs and requirements.

For following a liver detox diet, you have to know about your food options. From breakfast to daily snacks, everything is well-defined and structured in a way that you shed pounds fast and reverse fatty liver without compromising your health.

Chapter Twelve

Beginning a Fatty Liver Detox

To help you reverse fatty liver and restore health, a diet plan with some suitable recipes will be discussed in this chapter.

Before moving towards the proper diet plan during a liver detox, it is important to acknowledge the importance of drinking water. During your entire cleansing program, make your habit to drink two large glasses full of purified water. Add a bit of freshly squeezed lemon juice or grapefruit juice. If you have time, consider making fresh juice using raw vegetables including parsley, celery, and carrot.

Breakfast

For breakfast, consider any of the following food items:

- 2 to 4 eggs, preferably poached, scrambled, hard-boiled, or in the form of an omelet

- No Gran High Protein Muesli with low carbohydrates (recipe discussed later)

- Biodynamic acidophilus yogurt with no added flavor. Combine it with a pinch of stevia powder and a piece of fresh fruit.

- Fresh fruit salad with a few raw seeds and nuts

- Protein powder smoothie

- If you do not particularly feel hungry, rely on vegetable juice and a handful of seeds and nuts

It is extremely important to add fruits or vegetables in raw forms every day in your breakfast recipe. The preferred choices include pears, oranges, kiwi fruit, pineapple, cantaloupe, apples, melon, grapefruit, and pawpaw. Berries of all kinds including blueberries, plums, and strawberries are advised as they have slimming effects.

A no grain, high protein breakfast cereal is recommended to use for breakfast. You can easily make this at home using the following recipe.

Ingredients:

Equal parts of –

- Linseeds

- Sunflower seeds

- Hemp seeds
- Almonds
- Whey protein powder
- Psyllium husks

Start off by grinding all the seeds along with almonds in a food processor. The ground material can then be mixed in milk, most preferably coconut milk, rice milk, goat milk or organic cow milk. Plain yogurt can also be used instead of milk.

Lunch and Dinner

For lunch and dinner, you can choose any of the recipes that are discussed in this chapter. You can also just have a vegetable salad with a dressing made using lemon juice, cold-pressed oil, apple cider vinegar, or lime juice. Any cooked vegetables, including both green and starchy vegetables like sweet potato, parsnip, carrot, and pumpkin, can be included.

Lunch Ideas

Following are some of the lunch ideas that you may consider during a detox:

- Salad containing cherry tomatoes, feta cheese, olives, avocado, and green herbs such as basil.

- Traditional chicken soup

- Salad and a can of oily fish such as sardines, salmon, tuna, or mackerel.

- Gluten-free bread with red onions, avocados, olive oil, garlic, chopped tomatoes

- Grilled chicken breast along with sliced avocados, salad, and your favorite dressing

- Stir fry vegetables with soup

- Grilled fish with salad

- Sticks of fresh fruits, vegetables, cheese, and raw nuts dipped in hummus

Egg Fried Rice with Vegetables

Fried rice with vegetables and eggs serves as a delicious dinner while keeping low on bad nutrients side by side. To make this dish, the following items would be required.

- 2 beaten eggs

- 1tbsp of chili sauce

- Half a cup of chopped broccoli

- One-fourth cup of fresh basil leaves

- One-fourth tsp of stevia powder

- A clove of garlic in minced form

- 2 tbsp of olive oil

- 4 chopped scallions

- 10 sprigs of Cilantro

- Half a cup of shredded Chinese cabbage

- 1 cup of peas
- Sliced red bell pepper
- One and a half cups of brown, pre-cooked rice
- Half a cup of Mung bean sprouts
- 3 tbsp of soy sauce
- 1 stick of celery

Steam red bell peppers, cabbage, broccoli, and peas for about 2 minutes. Sauté scallions in oil for three minutes and add basil, cilantro, garlic, chili sauce, soy sauce, and sweetener. Now, add the pre-cooked rice along with the beaten eggs and stir. Add celery and bean sprouts at the end and stir it continuously until properly mixed and cooked.

Chili and Lime Fish

This recipe requires the following materials:

- 2 tbsp of olive oil
- 1 tbsp of fish sauce
- 2 tbsp of grated ginger
- 2 tbsp of lime juice
- 2 cloves of garlic, crushed properly
- Baby bok choys, 2 bunches
- 2 tbsp of sweet chili sauce
- 4 washed fillets of fish (as per your choice)

- Steamed jasmine rice
- 1 cup of cilantro leaves

Mix together oil, chili sauce, ginger, lime juice, fish sauce, and garlic. Add 2tbsp of all the ingredients instead of bok choys into a wok and boil it. Now add bok choys and cook the mixture for some time. Stir until the leaves obtain a bright green color and the stalks become tender. This will take about 2 minutes after which remove it from the stove. Brush the fish fillets using some lime juice. Grill both sides for 2 to 3 minutes. Place the cooked fish on rice and sprinkle some cilantro leaves on the top. Place some bok choys beside rice as well.

Roasted Vegetables

The ingredients required to prepare roast vegetables are:
- 1 leek
- 2 parsnips
- 1 brown onion
- 1 large-sized turnip
- 1 sweet potato of large size
- 3 carrots
- 2 bay leaves
- 2 sprigs of fresh and finely chopped rosemary
- 1 tbsp of soy sauce
- 1 tbsp of thyme

- 1 tbsp of mixed spices
- Black pepper
- Sea salt
- 2 tbsp of coconut oil

Cut all vegetables into thick strips like large potato wedges, except onion and leek. Slice onion into medium slices and leek into large pieces. In a large baking dish, put oil and tamari and put all the vegetables. Now add all the spices and put the covered dish in the oven to get baked. Wait for 30 minutes. Now remove the dish, stir, and place it back into the oven for an additional half-hour. Remove when the color turns brown and enjoy.

Chapter Thirteen

Salads to Detox Fatty Liver

Spinach Salad

What you need:

- A bunch of spinach
- 2 tbsp of virgin olive oil
- 2 tbsp of sesame seeds
- 1 tsp of soy sauce
- Macadamia oil
- 1 tbsp of freshly squeezed lemon juice
- A dash of sambal olek (tabasco)
- 8 fresh mushrooms in sliced form
- S50 grams if water chestnuts
- Chili paste (optional)

Remove and wash the spinach stems. Use a clean tea towel to dry them and put them in the refrigerator to crisp. Place sesame seeds in a pan and toast them. Remove it from the pan after a while. For salad dressing, mix lemon juice, oil, Tabasco, and soy sauce. Place the spinach leaves along with mushrooms and water chestnuts in a bowl and add sesame seeds. Now coat with salad dressing to finalize.

Beet Salad

What you need:

- 250 grams of steamed beets with skin removed
- 4 tbsp of virgin olive oil
- 3 tbsp of chopped cilantro leaves
- 3 tbsp of chopped red onion
- 2 tbsp of chopped mint leaves
- Freshly squeezed lemon juice (to taste)
- 1 tbsp of macadamia oil
- Half a cup of roasted walnuts
- Sea salt and pepper to taste
- 2 tbsp of rosewater
- Spinach leaves

Chop the beets into moderate-sized chunks while these are still warm. Mix the pieces with onions, cilantro, and other herbs. Whisk together lemon juice and oil in a bowl and add salt and pepper. Mix the ingredients with the dressing. Sprinkle some rose water right before serving.

Mushroom and Avocado Salad

What you need:

- 1 large avocado chopped into pieces
- 175 grams of fresh mushrooms, marinated
- 3 oranges, chopped
- 2 tbsp of freshly squeezed lemon juice
- 1 iceberg lettuce in chopped form
- 5 tbsp of orange juice
- 1 pinch of sea salt
- 1 tbsp of grated lemon zest
- 1 tbsp finely grated lemon zest
- 1 pinch sea salt
- Freshly ground black pepper

Mix lemon zest, orange juice, salt, and pepper in a bowl. Add the mushrooms to this mixture and let it stand for at least one hour. Now in a separate bowl, mix lemon juice, oranges, and avocados. Toss in some lettuce and the marinated mushrooms and enjoy the salad.

Marinated Vegetarian Asian-style Salad

What you need:

- 2 cloves of garlic, properly crushed
- 1 tbsp of sesame oil
- 1 tbsp of grated ginger
- One-fourth cup of soy sauce
- 500 grams of tempeh or bocconcini in sliced form
- 2 cups of red cabbage and shredded Chinese cabbage each
- 2 cups of bean sprouts
- Half a bunch of cilantro leaves
- Half a bunch of mint leaves
- Lime juice
- 2 finely sliced scallions
- 1 big carrot in a finely grated form
- A cup of grated daikon radish
- 1 tsp of sesame seeds

For Dressing:

- 2 tsp of sesame oil
- Lime juice
- 1 tbsp of soy sauce

- 2 tbsp of coconut oil
- 2 tbsp of sesame oil

For the marinade, mix tamari, ginger, garlic and sesame oil in a flat ceramic dish. Place the tempeh into the marinade and let it stay overnight. For the dressing, mix all the ingredients in a bowl, mix, and set aside. Take another bowl and mix the rest of the ingredients. Now put the prepared dressing into this bowl and toss them properly to coat the vegetables. Lastly, add the tempeh and mix well. Sprinkle some sesame seeds before serving.

Salad Dressings

For your convenience, ideas for making different salad dressings are included.

Salad Dressing 1

- Juice squeezed from 2 lemons
- 1 tbsp of honey
- 2 to 3 tbsp of olive oil
- 2 tsp of grainy mustard

Store it in a jar

Salad Dressing 2

- 1 tbsp of soy sauce
- Half a cup of balsamic vinegar

- Half a cup of olive oil
- 1 to 2 tsp of dried herbs

Place all the ingredients in a jar and shake it. Now store in a refrigerator.

Salad Dressing 3

- 1 tbsp of fresh garlic, peeled and crushed
- Half a cup of sesame oil
- Half a cup of olive oil
- Half tsp of dried cumin

Mix all the ingredients by placing the dressing in a jar and shaking it. Store in a refrigerator.

Salad Dressing 4

- Half a cup of lemon/orange juice
- Half a cup of natural yogurt
- 1 tbsp of chopped mint

Mix as per requirement

Hummus

What you require

- 400 grams of canned/ cooked chickpeas, properly rinsed
- A clove of garlic (crushed)
- Lemon juice to taste

- 3 tbsp of tahini

Mix all the ingredients together in a blender and enjoy.

Chapter Fourteen

Detox Soups for Fatty Liver

Liver Cleansing Soup

What you require

- 8 cups of water
- 2-3 fresh artichoke hearts (if available)
- 2 to 3 tbsp of olive oil (cold-pressed)
- 2 chopped potatoes
- 2 chopped celery
- 3 chopped tomatoes
- 2 chopped carrots
- 2 chopped beets
- 1 big red onion, chopped into small pieces
- 1 peeled and finely chopped ginger

- 1 clove of garlic (minced)
- 2 cups of sliced mushrooms
- 1 bunch of sliced bok choy
- One-fourth cup of arame seaweed in chopped form
- 1 cup of cooked beans or any lentils

Add celery seed, sea salt, turmeric, pepper and tamari to taste.

Add oil to a large saucepan and bring it to high heat. Now add tomato, ginger, celery, turmeric, onions, beets, potatoes, carrots, garlic, pepper, and some celery seeds. Mix the vegetables constantly to stop them from sticking to the ground. Now add water to the mixture and heat it up until it boils. Reduce the heat and let the solution simmer. Add mushrooms, seaweed, lentils, and artichoke hearts and mix. Let it simmer for 2 hours. Add bok choys to the soup sometime before serving. Throw in some tamari to taste.

Lentil Soup

What you require:

- Half a cup red lentils
- 1 cup of brown lentils
- 1 tsp of dried thyme
- 2 tsp of soy sauce
- 1 tsp of dried oregano

- Half a tsp of chili powder
- A handful of fresh basils in chopped form
- 2 chopped tomatoes
- 2 cups of chopped broccoli
- 2 sticks of finely chopped celery
- A handful of freshly chopped parsley
- 2 medium-sized brown onions, chopped
- A sprig of finely chopped rosemary
- 6 cups of water
- 2 tbsp of virgin olive oil
- 1 big leek in chopped form
- Ground pepper and sea salt
- 2 chopped carrots
- A few bay leaves
- Stock cube (optional)

Add some oil to the pan and fry the lentils on a low heat for 2 minutes. Now add garlic, onions, and tomatoes and cook for 3 more minutes. Add all the herb except parsley and keep cooking. Add the liquids, bay leaves, and a stock cube. Let the mixture simmer for 10 minutes. Add leek, celery, and carrot and let it stay on flames for an hour. In the last 20 minutes, add broccoli. Finish off by garnishing with parsley and parmesan.

Tomato Soup

- 6 chopped tomatoes
- 2 cloves of garlic
- 1 big onion
- 3 tbsp of olive oil
- Half a bunch of fresh basil leave
- 2 large-sized potatoes in the chopped form
- 2 cups of vegetable stock
- Black pepper and sea salt
- Grated parmesan cheese

Put all the ingredients in a baking pan except parmesan cheese. Bake until the vegetables become tender. Now place all the ingredients in a saucepan and cook for some time. Serve with parmesan.

Traditional Chicken Soup

To make traditional chicken soup, it is important to make a stock

- Free-range chicken
- A few bay leaves
- 1 cup of celery tops
- 1 large-sized onion, chopped
- Half a cup of parsley

- 2 cloves of garlic

Simmer the chicken for at least 90 minutes along with garlic, celery, onions, bay leaves, and parsley. Also, add 1.5 liters of water. Strain the mixture into a soup pot and keep it in the fridge overnight.

To make chicken soup, the following things will be required:

- 2 diced onions
- Half a bunch of fresh basil
- Some fresh cilantro
- 2 finely chopped carrots
- 6 stalks of celery, finely chopped
- 1 small-sized parsnip in chopped form
- 1 cup of chopped parsley
- 2 bay leaves
- 2 cups of water along with the vegetable stock cube
- Black pepper in ground form
- Sea salt to taste

Put onions, cilantro, basil, and parsley in a blender and process it. Cut chicken to form small cubes. Keep some of its large bones aside. Skim off the fat from the top of the stock. Take a large soup pot and place chicken bones, chicken pieces, and stock in it. Cover the pot and simmer it for 5 minutes. Add all the herbs and vegetables to the pot and cover it again. Let it simmer for 2 hours. Season the soup with black pepper and sea salt.

Chapter Fifteen

Other Foods for Fatty Liver Detox

Quick Snacks

• A protein smoothie made from a protein powder, coconut milk, and berries

• Sardines, crab meat, mackerel, salmon, or tuna. Mix it with 1 tbsp of fresh lime water and mayonnaise. Add herbs in chopped form and 2 rice thins

• Plain acidophilus yogurt. Make sure that there is no natural or artificial sugar added in it. You can consume about up to one cup of yogurt depending upon hunger. A piece of fresh fruit can be consumed with it.

• 1 to 2 pieces of raw fruit can be combined with raw nuts or 30 grams of cheese

• 50 to 60 grams of cheese. Choose from ricotta, vintage, feta, or plain cottage cheese. You can eat sticks of celery, carrot, capsicum, 4 sun-dried tomatoes, or 10 olives along with it

• Raw vegetable juice

• A handful of raw seeds and nuts of any variety. Salt can be added according to taste and a piece of fruit can be consumed with it.

• Raw vegetables, specifically carrot, zucchini, celery sticks, cucumber, broccoli florets, or snow peas dipped in hummus, tahini, bean dip, or avocado dip.

Low-Carbohydrate Ice-cream

To make the liver cleansing diet less boring, you can consider treating yourself with some low-carb ice cream from time to time. The following ingredients would be required to make it:

• 400 ml of fresh dairy cream

• 400 ml of coconut cream

• 2 tbsp of fresh fruits or frozen berries

• Half teaspoon of vanilla essence

• 2 tbsp of xylitol natural sweetener

Mix together dairy cream, sweetener, coconut cream and vanilla essence with the help of an electric beater. Throw in some fruits or berries of your choice. Now put the mixture in a flat container and wrap it up. Freeze it until it gets firm around the edges. Break the mixture and put it in a bowl. Use the beater again to make it smooth and creamy. Place the mixture back in the refrigerator until it sets. Serve in the form of scoops.

Raw Juices

Prepare and drink fresh juices on a daily basis during the entire length of liver cleanse. If you don't have time to prepare them on a daily basis, prepare it once a week and store it in glass jars. Include both fruits and vegetables that are fresh and in season.

Wash all the fruits or vegetables thoroughly and remove any blemished, bruised or moldy parts. Don't forget to include the leaves and stems of the vegetables while preparing juice as these parts are particularly high in minerals and vitamins.

If you observe that you are losing weight, do not include fruit juices in more than 10 percent recipes. Remember that vegetable juices have a lesser amount of carbohydrates and calories as compared to fruit juices and are, therefore, preferred.

Following are some of the recipes of juices that may help you to reverse fatty liver effectively.

Liver Cleansing Juice

What you require:

- 2 large-sized Brussels sprouts
- 2 large cabbage leaves or spinach
- Broccoli florets

- A clove of garlic
- Half cup of chopped parsley
- 1 whole apple

Wash all the ingredients thoroughly and chop them into small pieces. Process them into a juicer. The final mixture can be diluted with cold herbal tea or water in an equal ratio. Add grapes, beets, carrots or some strawberries to sweeten the taste.

Liver Tonic Juice

What you require:

- 130 grams of asparagus
- 130 grams of unpeeled cucumber
- 1 apple
- 1 carrot
- 2 leaves of cabbage

Wash and cut all the ingredients and toss them into the juicer for processing.

Fatty Liver Juice

What you require:

- Half cup of chopped parsley
- 2 carrots
- 1 red radish
- 1 clove of garlic

- 2.5 cm slice of fennel

- 1 lemon

- 2 cabbage leaves

- Red onion

Wash, cut and properly chop all the ingredients and mix it in the blender to form juice. This juice can be too strong for you. So, add 1 to 2 oranges or apples in the ingredients to tone it down. You can also add honey flavored tea, ginger, or a cup of cold lemon for added flavor.

Tips to Dine Out

Eating out is fun and cannot be cut out of life even if you are on detox. Therefore it is important to know about your possible options while you are dining out casually.

Thai, Chinese, and Vietnamese Cuisine

Try ordering their soups, salads, coconut dishes, rice, fresh rice paper rolls, or bean noodle dishes. Additionally, you can also rely on stir-fries such as Pad Thai or classic Vietnamese Pho. Asian seafood and green papaya salads can also be of great help.

Italian Cuisine

While in an Italian restaurant, strictly avoid consuming creamy pasta or pizzas of any kind. Instead, order polenta, lentil dishes, fish, vegetables, seafood risottos, salads, and soups. Salad dressings can be chosen in case they are free of sugar.

French Cuisine

Try your best to avoid pastries, white bread, creamy soups, and quiches. Soups that have flour added in them for thickness are also not recommended. Steer clear of rich desserts.

Japanese Cuisine

Try eating sashimi or sushi. Rice noodle dishes and ramen soups are also good options. Some Japanese restaurants also offer brown rice sushi rolls. Try these rolls along with salmon, tuna, cucumber, or avocado. You can also try brown rice sushi roll with miso soup for lunch. Stay away from tempura, meats coated with breadcrumb, and other deep-fried dishes.

Middle-Eastern Cuisine

Restrict yourself from pita, couscous, or Lebanese bread. Try having a falafel salad with baba ganoush dips or hummus on the side.

Indian Cuisine

Remember that chapattis and naan are not allowed during a liver cleanse. This also goes for all the deep-fried dishes. Eat lentils, vegetables, and dishes containing tofu or coconut spiced with curry, turmeric, and chili.

Café Cuisines

While dining out in a café, go for a Caesar salad with no added croutons. You can also order lentil salad, Nicoise salad, or salad containing prawns or other seafood. Omelets and scrambled eggs along with grilled vegetables are also good options. If you are craving for dessert, go for a gelato or sorbet ice cream instead of soft-serve ice cream. Yogurt or salad with fresh fruits can also make good desserts.

Detox Super Foods

While detoxing your liver, try including some exclusive foods in your everyday routine. These superfoods are important for getting an extra boost and are summarized below:

• Broccoli, cauliflower, Brussels sprouts, broccolini, red cabbage, watercress, and white cabbage

• Olives, garlic, parsley, globe artichokes, leeks, turmeric, scallions, ginger, and onions

• Bitter greens such as endive, radicchio, chicory, and rocket

• Bok choy, mustard greens, choy sum, and cilantro

• Fruits such as blueberries, apples, citrus fruits, and strawberries

• Seaweeds including wakame, kombu, nori, dulse, arame, and kelp. These can be used in salads, casseroles, stews, and soups

• Celery, carrots, asparagus, white daikon radish, and red radish

• Herbal teas made from peppermint, licorice, dandelion, peppermint, fennel, burdock, calendula, rooibos, ginger, or rosehip.

• Super greens including broccoli sprout powder, wheatgrass, barley grass, chlorella, and spirulina.

Chapter Sixteen

Simplifying your Fatty Liver Diet

Prohibited Foods

•   All types of preserved meats such as hot dogs, bacon, ham, and pepperoni. Canned meats, sausages, and pork are also restricted.

•   Processed oils and fats including canola, margarine, peanut oil, processed vegetable oil, palm oil, and corn oil are prohibited.

•   Caffeine-containing drinks like tea, coffee, and energy drinks. Green tea is an exception.

•   Processed foods must be avoided as they consist of hydrogenated fats, preservatives, sugar, and additives.

•   Do not use pesticides, insecticides or solvents with toxic chemicals.

- Fast foods of all types. Deep-fried dishes are also not allowed.

- Sugary drinks and sodas.

- Products containing white flour are prohibited.

- It is also important to stay away from alcohol, cigarettes, and recreational drugs during the entire duration of liver cleanse.

Shopping Tips

When you go shopping, make sure you keep in mind the following tips:

- Buy any kind of fruits but put special emphasis on buying citrus, berries, and avocado

- By any kind of vegetables as all of them are equally healthy

- Don't forget to buy brown rice

- Make sure to buy canned seafood like salmon, tuna, sardines, mackerel or trout

- Fresh seafood like lobster, crab, prawns, and calamari can also be bought

- Make sure buy organic chicken only

- Don't buy farmed eggs

- Lentils, chickpeas, and beans can also be bought

- For salad dressing make sure to buy apple cider vinegar

- Avoid garlic from the market, try to grow your own garlic

- Keep in mind to buy bowel cleansing powder like FiberTone

- Tamari, miso and soy sauce can also be bought

- Don't forget to buy nut butter like peanut butter, almond butter, hazelnut butter, cashew butter

- Grab that curry powder, ground turmeric, and cumin, caraway, fennel seeds.

- Make sure to buy dried seaweeds like nori, kombu, arame, dulse, and wakame

- Don't forget to buy LSA (Ground linseed, sunflower seeds, and almonds)

- In teas, you are free to buy green tea, black tea, licorice, peppermint, chamomile, dandelion, ginger tea, and rooibos.

- In the raw nuts portion, you are free to buy almonds, walnuts, Brazil, cashews, pine nuts, flax seeds, sunflower seeds, and hemp.

Vital Principles you Should Never Forget

Eat Raw

Thinking raw is one of the important things you should do to cleanse your liver effectively. Eat plentiful amounts of raw fruits like fruits and dark green leafy vegetables. Fruits which are orange, yellow, purple and red in color should never be ignored. It must be noted here that almost 40% of your diet must contain raw fruits and vegetables. Make sure that you eat any raw fruit or vegetable with every meal as they contain living enzymes, vitamin C, natural antibiotic substances and even anti-cancerous phytochemicals which, otherwise, can be damaged during cooking.

Don't load Up on Oil

Stay away from foods that present a high workload for your liver and gallbladder. Try to avoid margarine, processed vegetables, deep-fried foods, foods kept for more than 2 days as they contain rancid fats, preserved meats, and meats from very fat cattle. Always choose lean meat over fatty meat. Prevent yourself from buying creams, ice-creams, and processed cheeses. Obviously, fats are a vital part of your diet, therefore try to eat healthy fats which are found in commonly occurring foods like olive oil, avocados, fish (especially that of salmon, tuna, sardines, herring, cod, flounder, bass and mackerel), raw seeds (specially of linseeds, sunflower seeds, sesame seeds hemp seeds, alfalfa seeds, pumpkin seeds and legumes) and raw fresh nuts. If you are not easy with eating whole seed, you can grind them fresh every day in a regular coffee grinder or any common food processor. This ground material can be put into cereals, smoothies, fruit salads, and even vegetables. Make sure you don't use margarine on your bread or even crackers.

Recipe: If you still crave for margarine, alternatively use tahini, hummus, pesto, tomato paste or freshly ground garlic and cold-pressed oil. You can also add some chilies or other spices to make it more enjoyable.

The use of margarine with crackers or bread is not healthy. If you really crave it, try using hummus, tahini, tomato paste, pesto or a combination of cold-pressed liver and fresh garlic in minced form. Spices such as chili can also be added to taste. You can also try eating nut spreads for the same purpose. Butter can be used as a spread but keep in mind to spread it in the form of a thin layer. Observing a liver cleanse does not mean to cut off the fat intake entirely. Remember that good fats play a crucial role in building the cell membranes of the liver cells. As you age, the requirement of the body for oil increases, but this does not mean greasing it up.

Prefer the Naturals

This is a particularly important step to observe during a liver cleanse. Steer clear of all the artificially created toxins and chemicals. This includes artificial sweeteners, pesticides, and insecticides. Aspartame is an artificial sweetener that is not to be used under any circumstances. While choosing your cosmetics, prefer those that are close to the natural forms and are free of excessive chemicals.

Observe Diversity

Be sure to observe diversity in terms of proteins. Use everything, starting from raw nuts, legumes, and seeds to eggs, cheese, plain yogurt, lean fresh red meat, chicken meat, and seafood. If you are not a fan of poultry or red meat, there is no need to worry as there are a lot of other protein sources. You can also be a strict vegetarian if you like, however, this will require you to take additional supplements of iron, vitamin B12, glutamine, and taurine to prevent the weakening of the immune system and other problems such as anemia.

To obtain the first-class protein through diet, the vegetarians have to combine 3 out of the following 4 classes of food during one meal:

- Nuts
- Grains
- Legumes
- Seeds

If this is not observed, there might be deficiencies seen in the concentration of essential amino acids in your body. A lack of amino acids will then allow you to suffer from fatigue and frequent mood swings. Your cognitive function will be reduced, the immune system will weaken, hypoglycemia will prevail and the liver function will suffer from further disturbance. In my life, I have come across a lot of vegetarians who always felt unwell because their body lacked in amino acids, vitamin B12 or iron. By supplementing their bodies with these nutrients and changing their dietary plans, a significant level of improvement was observed.

Make Food your Medicine

Carefully follow the optimal dietary habits and amaze yourself with the strong healing power of foods. In addition to fatty liver, several other diseases can also be overcome by just changing your diet plan and eating foods that possess strong medicinal features. Ensuring to eat such foods can not only treat the diseases but can also prevent its recurrences. The culinary habits belonging to different cultures have also been recognized to have a special influence on the incidence of diseases and the total lifespan. An example of this is the Mediterranean diet which has been previously discussed to play a significant role in the reversal of fatty liver.

In the case of liver-related problems, foods such as turmeric, milk thistle, globe artichoke, and dandelion are of particular importance. Moreover, natural sources of antioxidants like selenium, vitamin E, carotenoids, and vitamin C are also appreciable. Relying on foods that have high levels of sulfur-containing amino acids such as glutamine, taurine, glutathione, glycine, methionine, and cysteine can also cure liver diseases. The sulfurated phytochemicals often found in cruciferous vegetables also mimic the medicines in providing relief from liver diseases such as fatty liver.

Broccoli and other vegetables belonging to the cruciferous family are famous for their effects to prevent the incidence of bowel cancer as well. Broccoli consists of a phytochemical known as sulforaphane. This phytochemical is of particular importance during phase 2 of detoxification pathway occurring in the liver. Tomato is an important dietary item that is loaded with a powerful antioxidant known as lycopene. Researchers have regarded it as the most powerful of all the carotenoids naturally occurring in food. Cooking tomato increases the absorption level of lycopene whereas eating a tomato with oil enhances the availability of this carotenoid in the body.

The beautiful purple color of beets is because of the presence of anthocyanidin, a powerful antioxidant. The constituents of beets have been indicated to be of particular benefits to the body, mimicking the effects of drugs. Other food items that are proven to provide similar effects include cranberries, red onions, red bell peppers, turmeric, and paprika. These foods have high concentrations of certain healing phytonutrients including capsanthin, Curcumin, and anthocyanins.

The Mediterranean and the Asian cuisines are now integrating themselves into the Western diet that comprises of bread, meat, and four vegetables. This multiculturalism in terms of culinary aspects has proven to be extremely beneficial for health as well as for enjoyment. It is rightly said that variety is the spice of life, and the incorporation of Mediterranean and Asian foods in the Western culture has added a little spice to the typical bland ways of eating. The vegetables and foods included in the typical Asian culture such as chili, ginger, garlic, bok choy, Chinese water spinach, turmeric, lemongrass, Chinese mushrooms, curry, and other items can be experimented with and introduced into the daily routine of meals in order to enjoy new tastes as you improve your health.

Say No to Sugars

Saying no to sugar does not mean you should be completely cutting it off your life. Instead, try switching to natural sugars found in fresh fruits. You can also use honey, dried fruits, fruit sorbets, carob, fruit jams, maple syrup, molasses, and date sugar in small amounts

Things you should be saying no to include lollies, white refined sugar, cakes, fizzy drinks, and cookies made using refined sugar. Excessive use of these food items can further exacerbate the condition of the fatty liver and may also increase its chances of recurrence even if treated properly. Keep in mind that an excessive amount of carbohydrates and natural sugars are converted into fat eventually. Eat more protein and treat yourself to nutrients such as magnesium and chromium as it will get your craving under control and sufficiently aid you in losing weight and shedding the fat surrounding your liver. Apple cider vinegar and cinnamon can also be used to reduce cravings.

Keep the Body Hydrated

Rely on a lot of fluids including teas, raw vegetable juices, and of course, water. You can use herbal tea, green tea, and even regular black tea for this purpose. Set your goal to consume at least 70oz or 2 liters of fluid in any form on a daily basis. This will ensure that constipation remains at distance and the toxins that have been broken down by the liver are properly excreted via the kidneys.

Consider installing a household water filter. Go for water filters that have sub-micron, solid carbon block filters as they can effectively remove different parasites and other toxic materials from the body. Shop around and take your time looking at different varieties of filters before choosing one. It is also advised to get the help of a professional because of the rapid advancements in the technological area.

It is basically the function of a liver to detoxify the body and get rid of harmful materials. However, it is necessary to support its functions with the help of other body organs. The kidneys and the skin are of particular importance in this regard and can support the liver by getting rid of the toxins through urination and sweating. This is the reason why a high water intake and saunas can efficiently reduce the signs of toxic overload.

Be Organic

It is always the ideal option to buy organic products from the market and use it. However, this might not be suitable in terms of logistical or financial reasons. You do not need to take stress because even if the diet that you are taking is not organic, it is still healthy and extremely important for health.

No one wants to consume fruits and vegetables that have been repeatedly exposed to protective chemical sprays such as fungicides and insecticides, ripened using ethylene gas, or simply waxed by the secretion of an insect. It is unpleasant as you bite off a piece of your delicious steak that this animal might have been fed the remains of thousands of dead animals and other chemical agents such as antibiotics. It might have been implanted with growth hormones just to fasten up his speed of growth as well.

The general "healthy" reputation of beef was destroyed particularly after the prevalence of mad cow disease, a problem that has been disturbing England for quite some time now. In the year 1996, the government of Britain disclosed how the mad cow disease had a tendency to pass to the human race in the form of a fatal disease known as Creutzfeldt Jakob Disease. It has also been discovered that a different form of Creutzfeldt Jakob Disease can also be manifested in pigs and chicken and the disease might not be able to manifest itself completely because of the slaughtering of these animals before they fully develop. For this purpose, the government has banned the farmers from feeding dead cattle to the livestock. The opinions regarding the cause of mad cow disease and Creutzfeldt Jakob Disease since it is quite difficult to assess them in the infected animals. Because of this reason, a worldwide ban on feeding livestock with animal tissue must be banned as per WHO.

Organic food is also known as biodynamic food sometimes and is produced without the use of any synthetic herbicides, fertilizers, insecticides, and post-harvest fungicides. Moreover, the complete prohibition of hormones to promote growth or enhance size is strictly observed. Organic food completely relies on the force of Mother Nature, sustainable production methods, and nutrient recycling for this purpose. Such type of food has to be grown n farms which are continuously inspected and have full certification as per the set standards. The processed or packaged organic foods are completely free of any type of preservatives, flavors, colorings, or additives. Such types of food also do not contain any genetically modified or irradiated ingredients. The best idea for getting organic food is to pot plants or grow fruits, vegetables, and herbs in your backyard.

Maintain the Health of Your Bowel

Maintain the health of your bowel and keep it safe from developing constipation by eating a lot of fiber. Fiber can be easily found in raw forms of fruits and vegetables and all unprocessed foods. Another good way to prevent constipation is to make a natural medicine by yourself. Grind flaxseeds, almonds, and sunflower seeds in a blender to form a fine powder. You can also use other seeds to make this powder. Pumpkin seeds, psyllium, and sesame seeds are particularly high in fiber and can be a great addition to the powder.

Consume up to 3 tablespoons of this powder on a daily basis to upkeep your bowel health. In addition to consuming directly, you can also add the powder to soups, smoothies, fruit salads, and cereals to enjoy its benefits.

Fiber works like a broom within your bowls, sweeping all the harmful and waste materials. It has the power to thoroughly clean the digestive system and excrete waste substances via bowel actions. So, adding fiber in your life is going to make you live a healthy life completely free of all kinds of diseases.

Be Selective

Being selective in terms of food is always wise. Always aim for the quality and the taste a particular food item has to offer instead of its quantity. Always be more conscious of what you eat. Take small bites and chew slowly and properly so that you can relish the taste of natural foods, spices, oils, and herbs. Do not eat more than you require and always keep your ears open to what your body might be trying to tell you.

Stop eating the moment you feel full. Overeating for a consistent amount of time will increase the workload on your liver and may also reduce its capacity to detoxify the body from harmful chemical materials. The overworked liver will also find it difficult to burn fat and you will be at an increased risk of developing a recurrent episode of fatty liver. Do not dig your own grave and eat healthy always.

Take Care of your Health

Try to eat food that provides your body with nutrients that particularly improve the function of your liver. Some of these nutrients include:

Vitamin K

Vitamin K can be taken from natural food sources, particularly fresh green herbs, green leafy vegetables, spirulina, asparagus, and cruciferous vegetables. Drinking juices of these green vegetables, particularly celery, kale, barley-grass, what grass, or mint.

Glutamine

Glutamine is an amino acid that helps in the detoxification of ammonia. Ammonia exists as a waste product in your body and can be toxic if not removed properly. Consuming food rich in glutamine can help in the removal of this substance. To consume glutamine, take it in powder form and combine it with cool beverages. Avoid mixing it in hot drinks as warmth can cause its denaturation. You can also take it in combination with selenium to improve the overall function of glutathione- one of the most powerful antioxidants of the liver.

Antioxidants

Antioxidants can be consumed from certain food items such as globe artichoke, milk thistle, dandelion, and turmeric. Fruits and vegetables are also a good source of these agents.

Selenium

Selenium itself possesses antioxidant properties and can be taken in the form of molasses, Brazil nuts, onions, garlic, wheat germ, seafood, and kelp. The amount of selenium carried by these food items depends upon the quality of soil in which they are being grown. Most parts of the world do not have the right kind of soil for these foods to develop enough selenium.

Methionine

Methionine is an extremely important amino acid for detoxification. It can be easily obtained in high levels from foods like fish, legumes, eggs, onions, garlic, and meat.

Essential Fatty Acids

The best sources to obtain all the essential fatty acids are cod liver oil, oily fish, and fish oil. Both fresh and canned seafood can be used for this purpose. Additionally, raw seeds and nuts, freshly ground seeds, eggplant, avocados, hemp seeds, and flaxseeds can also be of great help in this regard. Hemp seeds need not be ground. Essential fatty acids are essential because they improve liver function.

This is the reason why low-fat diets are generally not considered as healthy for weight control, liver health, and general body functions.

Natural Sulfur Compounds

Natural compounds of sulfur are basically found in free-range eggs and a variety of other food items such as leeks, garlic, scallions, onions and some cruciferous vegetables such as cauliflower, broccoli, Brussels sprouts, and cabbage.

Maintain Good Hygiene

One of the basic functions of the liver is to remove the microorganisms from the blood and prevent them from accessing the deeper portions of the body and causing diseases. In order to avoid the overloading of the liver, it is important that you avoid eating that has a high chance of being contaminated by unfriendly and potentially dangerous pathogens.

The standards of living have generally improved a lot. Yet, the causes of bacteria and viruses causing food poisoning in people have been on the rise. This is mostly because of poor hygienic measures such as improper cleaning of the areas where food is stored or cooked, and poor standards of handwashing, particularly before cooking and eating food.

The practice of poor hygiene has become more common these days as the people have been given false assurances by antibiotic drugs. However, many strains of drug-resistant pathogens have started to occur raising the concern of the people. People are also more likely to eat out and cook less at home, making it more difficult to control the standards of hygiene during food preparation.

People buy food items from supermarkets that have traveled long distances possibly in unfavorable conditions and are then stored for extended periods of time. This allows them to become an ideal habitat for microorganisms. A lot of foods contain preservatives for this purpose, however, most of the time, these preservatives do not have the ability to eradicate the microorganisms. Instead, these preservatives just keep them in a dormant form.

When such types of food contaminated with pathogens enter your body, the preservatives become diluted and fail to control the pathogens which rapidly start multiply. This is why it is important for you to buy fresh food of the highest quality. Remember that the risk of food contamination increases by several folds if the food is kept stored for a long period of time. Handling and packaging of food by multiple people and inadequate temperatures for cooling and heating can also be considered among the factors contributing to food contamination.

Tips to Maintain Hygiene

For a healthy liver, you need to observe good general health. Sanitation is necessary to observe good body health. Following techniques will make it easy for you to observe hygiene:

•   Use soap and warm water to thoroughly wash your hands before you start handling any raw food, especially seafood and meat. Brush under your nails using a nailbrush as this can get rid of all the bacteria which are not accessible through hand washing techniques. Also wash all the cutting boards, kitchen utensils, blenders, juicers, grinders, and can openers both before and after using them.

• Only buy fresh foods and avoid all the food items that look old or are moldy. Also stay away from preserved or processed foods such as ham, hamburger meat, pickled, and smoked meat. Other foods to avoid are sausages, bacon, beef jerky, cabanossi, meat patties, meatballs, pizza meats, rolled meats, and corned beef. Poorly stored or mishandled seafood is also not safe for use.

• Do not let the food items stand in hot temperatures for more than 2 hours.

Chapter Seventeen

Conclusion

Diets for fatty liver will continue to come and go. Some of them would indeed be dangerous and will definitely make you miserable because some of them are too restrictive while others are impractical and extremely hard to follow. There are a lot of diets that can reverse fatty liver and the key is to pick the one that suits you. A diet that will help you lose pounds while improving your body metabolism and strengthening your immune system is the key.

"There are currently no drugs on the market which are approved by the U.S FDA for fatty liver, therefore losing 10% of your body weight would be an ideal approach (even 3-5% can do the trick)."

By following a suitable diet plan, it is completely possible to reverse fatty liver. If you have been unfortunate enough to suffer from this disease, do not hassle. The ability of our body to survive, adapt, and thrive will always continue to amaze you. With proper nutrition and dietary patterns, your body can heal itself and reverse fatty liver and almost any other illness.

Many Blessings

Junaid Tariq

One last thing!

I want to give you a **one-in-two-hundred chance** to win a **$200.00 Amazon Gift card** as a thank-you for reading this book.

All I ask is that you give me some feedback, so I can improve this or my next book :)

Your opinion is *super valuable* to me. It will only take a minute of your time to let me know what you like and what you didn't like about this book. The hardest part is deciding how to spend the two hundred dollars! Just follow this link.

http://reviewers.win/fattyliver

www.ingramcontent.com/pod-product-compliance
Lightning Source LLC
Chambersburg PA
CBHW021442210526
45463CB00002B/613